CANCER SURVIVAL TIPS

A must know survival tips for people battling with cancer

Mr Marcus Baldwin

CONTENTS

INTRODUCTION

A group of diseases known as cancer are defined by the unchecked growth and division of abnormal cells. These cells can develop tumors or infiltrate other tissues and organs, which can result in a number of health concerns. People of all ages, races, and genders are susceptible to developing cancer, which can impact virtually any part of the body.

Cancer comes in a wide variety of forms, including breast cancer, colorectal cancer, lung cancer, prostate cancer, and many more. Genetics, environmental variables, and lifestyle choices like smoking, eating poorly, and not exercising are just a few of the causes of cancer.

Cancer signs and symptoms can differ depending on the type and stage of the disease, but some typical ones are unexplained weight loss, fatigue, pain, skin changes, and changes in bowel or bladder habits. It's important to talk with your healthcare practitioner if you have any unusual symptoms or health concerns.

Cancer treatment can involve surgery, radiation therapy, chemotherapy, immunotherapy, or a combination of these modalities depending on the type and stage of the illness. Although improvements in cancer care have improved many patients' results, the disease still poses a serious threat to global health. The risk of cancer can be decreased and general health can be improved with routine screenings and healthy lifestyle decisions.

Cancer is a condition that can be physically and psychologically taxing for both the sufferer and their loved ones. However, there are some survival strategies that can improve a person's odds of recovery while also assisting them in coping with cancer.

INCREASING POSITIVE EMOTIONS

A cancer diagnosis can be a difficult and difficult experience, and it is natural to feel a variety of emotions during this time. However, studies have shown that maintaining a positive attitude and increasing positive emotions can have a number of benefits for cancer patients.

Among the methods for boosting positive feelings and improving emotional well-being during cancer treatment are:

1.Practicing gratitude: Concentrating on the positive aspects of life and expressing gratitude for them can help to divert your attention away from negative thoughts and emotions.

2.Participating in enjoyable activities: Engaging in enjoyable activities, such as hobbies or spending time with loved ones, can help to boost mood and promote positive emotions.

3. Mindfulness techniques such as meditation or deep breathing exercises can help to reduce stress and increase feelings of calm and relaxation.

4. Building and keeping supportive relationships with family and friends can help to increase feelings of social support and decrease feelings of isolation.

5. Seeking professional help: Speaking with a mental health professional or joining a cancer support group can provide a secure and supportive environment for people to share their feelings and receive guidance and support.

While keeping a positive attitude can have many benefits for cancer patients, it is also important to remember that experiencing a range of feelings throughout the cancer journey is normal and healthy. When needed, it is critical to obtain support and care from a healthcare professional and loved ones.

RELEASING SUPPRESSED EMOTIONS

Cancer is a difficult and emotional journey, and it is normal to feel a variety of emotions during this time. Some people, however, may find themselves suppressing their emotions in order to deal with the stress and uncertainty that cancer brings. While this coping strategy may provide brief relief, suppressing emotions can have long-term negative consequences for both emotional and physical health.

Releasing suppressed emotions can help cancer patients manage and enhance their emotional well-being. Here are some methods that may be useful:

1. Journaling: Keeping a private diary and writing down thoughts and feelings can help you process emotions and gain insights into underlying feelings and beliefs.

2. Talking to an expert in mental wellness can help you express your feelings and work through your difficult cancer-related emotions in a safe and encouraging setting.

3. Art therapy: Expressing oneself through artistic endeavors like painting, sculpting, or drawing can help with emotional release.

4. Techniques for the mind-body connection: Activities

like yoga, tai chi, or guided meditation can ease tension and stress and encourage relaxation, which can help to open up previously repressed feelings.

5. Joining a support group can give you a sense of community, understanding, and a secure place to share your emotions. Connecting with others who have battled cancer can do the same.

It is crucial to keep in mind that releasing repressed feelings can be a gradual process, so one must be patient and kind to themselves. A crucial step in this process can be to ask for help and support from loved ones and medical professionals.

TAKING CONTROL OF YOUR HEALTH

It can be overwhelming to receive a cancer diagnosis, but there are things you can do to take charge of your health and enhance your general wellbeing while undergoing cancer therapy. Here are some tactics to take into account:

1. Learn more: Do as much research as you can on your cancer prognosis and available therapies. Ask your medical team questions and look for reliable sources of knowledge.

2. Maintain a healthy lifestyle: Eating a balanced diet, exercising frequently, and getting adequate rest can all support your body's healing from cancer therapy and enhance general health.

3. Promote your own interests: Ask for assistance when you require it and let your healthcare staff know your needs and preferences. Participate actively in your treatment choices and adhere to your treatment plan's instructions.

4. Manage stress: Develop coping mechanisms to deal with it, including relaxation exercises, enjoyable pursuits, and assistance from family members or a mental health expert.

5. Be organized: To make sure you are staying on top of your healthcare requirements, stay organized by keeping track of your doctor's appointments,

treatment plans, and medication schedules.

6. Join an advocacy group: Making connections with other cancer survivors can foster a sense of belonging and empathy and offer a secure setting for sharing feelings and experiences.

CANCERS WEAKNESSES

Cancerous cells have genetic mutations that make them proliferate and enlarge out of control. Despite the fact that cancer cells have a variety of characteristics that make them challenging to treat, there are some universal flaws that can be addressed in cancer treatment:

1. Rapid division: Since cancer cells reproduce much more quickly than healthy cells do, they need a lot of energy and nutrients to survive. By focusing on these metabolic weaknesses, their development can be slowed or stopped.

2. Tumors require blood flow to live and develop, which is known as angiogenesis. Drugs that prevent the formation of new blood vessels (angiogenesis) can slow the development of tumors.

3. DNA damage: Because of their rapid division and other factors, cancer cells have a high incidence of DNA damage. Cancer cells can be killed by drugs that particularly target damaged DNA.

4. Immune evasion: Cancer cells frequently evade the immune system, enabling them to grow unchecked. Immunotherapy drugs stimulate the immune system, causing it to identify and attack cancer cells.

5. Cell death resistance: Cancer cells have developed mechanisms to resist programmed cell death, also known as apoptosis. Cancer cells may die if these processes are targeted.

6. Inflammation: Inflammation can encourage cancer cell growth and spread. Anti-inflammatory drugs can slow or stop tumor development.

It's important to remember that cancer is a complex illness with numerous types and subtypes, and each cancer has its own set of vulnerabilities. As a result, the best method to target cancer cells will rely on the type of cancer and the characteristics of the cancer cells in each individual patient.

HERBS AND SUPPLEMENT USAGE

I must stress that using herbs and supplements to treat cancer is a complicated and debatable subject, so it's crucial to speak with a trained healthcare provider before utilizing any alternative therapies.

The efficacy and safety of many herbs and supplements for humans are still largely unknown, and many supplements can interact negatively with prescription medications. Nevertheless, some herbs and supplements have demonstrated encouraging results in laboratory studies and animal trials.

It's crucial to discuss any potential use of herbs and supplements with your doctor or another qualified healthcare provider because some supplements may even conflict with cancer therapy.
Working closely with your medical team is crucial to making sure that any herbs or vitamins you use are secure, efficient, and supportive of your cancer treatment strategy.

CANCER FIGHTING SURROUNDINGS

An "anti-cancer environment" is one that promotes a way of living and surroundings that help prevent or reduce the chance of developing cancer. Here are some ideas for creating an anti-cancer environment:

1. Develop a healthy weight: Obesity and being overweight have been related to a variety of cancers. A healthy diet and regular physical exercise can help you maintain a healthy weight and lower your risk of cancer.

2. Consume a healthy diet: Eating a diet rich in fruits, vegetables, whole grains, and lean protein can help lower the chance of cancer. It is also advised to avoid processed meals and foods rich in saturated and trans fats.

3. Stay away from tobacco: Tobacco use and smoking are the main causes of cancer. Tobacco and secondhand smoke avoidance can greatly reduce your cancer risk.

4. Minimize alcohol intake: Alcohol consumption raises the risk of several cancers, including breast, liver, and colorectal cancer. Drinking one drink per day for women and two drinks per day for males can help reduce cancer risk.

5. Safeguard your skin: The most prevalent form of cancer is skin cancer. Sunscreen, protective clothing, and avoiding midday sun exposure can all help to lower your risk.

6. remain active: Regular physical exercise can help lower your cancer risk. Aim for 150 minutes of moderate-intensity exercise per week or 75 minutes of vigorous-intensity exercise.

7. Vaccinate yourself: Certain viruses, such as HPV and hepatitis B, can increase your risk of developing certain kinds of cancer. Getting vaccinated against these viruses can help lower your chance of developing cancer.

8. Managing stress: Chronic stress can weaken the immune system and increase inflammation, increasing the chance of cancer. Stress-relieving pursuits such as meditation, yoga, or deep breathing can aid in stress management.

You can establish a cancer prevention environment for yourself and lower your risk of developing cancer by following these steps.

Every person's experience with cancer is different, so it's crucial to collaborate with your healthcare team to create a strategy that is specific to your requirements. Participating actively in your healthcare can enhance your general wellbeing while battling cancer.

ENHANCING YOUR SPIRITUALITY WHILE UNDERGOING ILLNESS

A cancer prognosis can be an extremely difficult and emotional experience, leading many people to look for spiritual support and direction. During cancer, try these strategies to strengthen your mental connection:

1. Meditation: Using this technique, you can calm your mind and develop a stronger feeling of inner calm and connection. Locate a peaceful area where you can relax and sit or lay down comfortably. Concentrate on your breathing or a particular mantra or phrase.

2. Prayer: Forging a connection with a higher force or a source of strength through prayer can be very effective. Whether you adhere to a particular religious practice or not, making time for prayer can be a source of solace and power.

3. Nature: Spending time in nature can be a powerful way to experience awe and wonder at the world around you. Walk through a park or relax outside while you take in the sounds of nature.

4. Spiritual community: Finding like-minded people to

connect with can be a great source of strength and solace. Attending religious events or affiliating with a spiritual movement or group is an option.

5. Expressing yourself creatively can be a great way to explore your faith and connect with your inner self. Examples of creative endeavors include writing, music, and art. Give yourself permission to feel what you are feeling and to connect with your inner knowledge.

CANCER FIGHTING FOODS

SCIENTIFICALLY PROVEN BEST FOODS FOR CANCER PATIENTS

The inevitable question: Are vegetarians more cancer-resistant just because they don't consume meat? Or is it the food they consume that is to blame?

It is true that plant-based foods, such as whole grains, legumes, nuts, and fruits and vegetables, are nutrient-dense. Additionally, studies have connected eating a lot of them to a decreased risk of cancer.

While no single food can cure cancer, a healthy and balanced diet can help prevent cancer and support cancer treatment. A diet high in fruits and vegetables, whole grains, and lean protein sources can help reduce cancer risk and improve overall health.

Furthermore, certain foods, such as cruciferous vegetables like broccoli and kale, berries like blueberries and strawberries, and fatty fish like salmon, have been shown to have anti-cancer properties. It should be noted, however, that relying solely on diet to treat cancer is ineffective, and a proper medical treatment plan should always be followed under the supervision of a healthcare professional.

As a result, while including healthy foods in your diet is certainly beneficial, it is not a replacement for medical treatment. To determine the best course of action for managing and treating cancer, it is critical to consult with a healthcare professional.

An elaboration: Plants create a large number of phytochemicals, or plant compounds, which may shield cells from harm. Phytochemicals offer a number of advantageous properties, such as being anti-inflammatory.

USE SMOOTHIES TO UP YOUR CALORIE AND NUTRIENT INTAKE.

Smoothies are a terrific way to consume more calories, protein, fiber, hydration, vitamins, and minerals. If you have mouth sores, they are also soothing. By including nut butters, avocado, plain Greek yogurt, flaxseed oil, or other healthy oils, you can increase the calorie content of smoothies. To increase nutrition and add flavor, you can include fresh or frozen fruits, berries, and a variety of liquid bases (almond milk, coconut water).

CANCER FIGHTING FROZEN DELIGHT

For cancer patients, particularly those who might be dealing with nausea or mouth sores as a result of treatment, there are a number of frozen treats that can be a cool and enjoyable choice. Here are some suggestions:

1. Fruit popsicles: Fruit popsicles, whether homemade or purchased from a shop, can be a refreshing and tasty treat. Choose products that are created with actual fruit and no additional sugar.

2. Fruit puree, sugar, and water are used to make the frozen treat sorbet. It can be a good alternative for people who are lactose intolerant or have digestive problems because it usually contains less fat than ice cream.

3. Frozen yogurt: Frozen yogurt is made with yogurt rather than cream and is comparable to ice cream. It may be simpler for some cancer patients to process because it has fewer calories and fat than ice cream.

4. Smoothies: These hydrating and nutrient-rich treats can be prepared with frozen fruit, yogurt, milk, or juice. To add more vitamins and minerals, try blending in some spinach or other leafy vegetables.

5. Fruit ice is a frozen treat prepared from fruit and sugar

syrup that is then frozen in a shallow dish. It has a fluffy, icy substance when scraped with a utensil.

Before making major dietary changes, always consult your physician or a registered dietitian, particularly if you are receiving treatment for cancer. Based on your particular requirements and treatment strategy, they can offer suggestions that are tailored to you.

A plant based diet can help lower your cancer risk
Most food that reduces your cancer risk is plant food that contains phytochemicals.

There have been studies and discoveries of more than 4,000 phytochemicals. There isn't a single superfood that has them all. They all have various advantages and purposes."

No single diet can prevent cancer, but the appropriate combination of meals can help. Aim for at least two-thirds plant-based foods and no more than one-third animal protein at mealtime. According to the American Institute for Cancer Research, this "New American Plate" is an essential cancer-fighting strategy. Examine the best and worst options for your plate.

There is no single food that can avoid or cure cancer, but certain foods are known to contain cancer-fighting nutrients. The following substances have been shown to have anti-cancer properties:

MEAT CONSUMPTION AND CANCER RATES

Meat lovers might be lured to eat their steak and a salad if it's all about consuming a lot of phytochemicals and fiber. Additionally, research points to a connection between meat and cancer.

Study found that the relative risk of colorectal polyps increased by 2% for every additional 3.5 ounces of red meat consumed daily. A daily intake of only half as much processed meat—such as deli meats or hot dogs—increased the risk by 29%.

So what's the issue with meat?

There is evidence that eating more of it increases the chance of death from any cause. A significant factor is that cooking red meat is thought to produce cancer-causing chemical components. Apparently helping are the compounds found in processed beef.

Your health will improve if you consume less red and processed meat. A decent rule of thumb is to eat no more than 12 to 18 ounces of red meat or processed meat each week if you don't want to go cold turkey. The weight of three ounces is comparable to the size of your palm.

THE ART OF BALANCING

It can be best to make modest changes if you want to transition to a more plant-based diet that you'll want to maintain. There are various techniques to use;

1. Try cooking vegetarian dishes. Make it a point to try one new meatless recipe each week. Alliteration is only one aspect of "Meatless Monday," though. Starting a new, healthy habit at the beginning of the week might increase your likelihood of success.

2. Use beans as a filler. Increase the amount of beans, lentils, or vegetables in several dishes to reduce the overall amount of meat. Additionally, because we frequently eat with our eyes and such things take up more space on your plate, you won't feel restricted.

3. Use meat as a garnish. Use some meat as flavoring rather than as the main course. To obtain the flavor in every mouthful without using much, you can cut turkey bacon into very little bits and sprinkle it over a pita pizza.

There are many different ways to eat a plant-based diet. Small adjustments can make a significant difference.

Eating particular meals won't make you less likely to develop cancer. However, you can significantly lower your risk if you concentrate on eating a plant-based diet and keeping a healthy weight.

1. Fruits and vegetables are high in antioxidants, which serve to protect cells from damage that can lead to

cancer. Cruciferous veggies like broccoli, cauliflower, and Brussels sprouts are especially nutritious.

2. Berries are high in polyphenols and other antioxidants that have been linked to anti-cancer qualities. Berries such as blueberries, raspberries, strawberries, and blackberries are all excellent options.

3. Garlic and onions: Sulfur compounds found in garlic and onions have been shown to have anti-cancer effects. It is best to consume these foods raw or lightly cooked to retain their cancer-fighting properties.

4. Turmeric: Curcumin, a compound found in turmeric, has been shown to have anti-inflammatory and anti-cancer effects. Including turmeric in your diet or taking a curcumin supplement can help enhance its anti-cancer properties.

5. Green tea includes catechins, which are antioxidants that have been shown to have anti-cancer properties. Green tea consumption on a regular basis can help safeguard cells from cancer-causing damage.

6. Nuts and seeds contain healthy fats, fiber, and antioxidants that can help safeguard cells from cancer-causing damage. Almonds, walnuts, chia seeds, and flaxseeds are all excellent sources of omega-3 fatty acids.

7. Whole grains contain fiber, vitamins, and minerals that can help lower the chance of several types of cancer. To boost your intake, choose whole grain bread, pasta, rice, and cereal.

Despite the fact that these foods have been shown to have anti-cancer qualities, it's critical to remember that they should be included in a healthy, balanced diet. A healthy weight and eating a range of foods are essential for lowering your risk of cancer.

CANCER FIGHTING WITH COLOUR

Cancer-preventing nutrients are abundant in fruits and vegetables, and the more color a food has, the more nutrition it has. When you achieve and keep a healthy body weight, these meals can also reduce your risk in another way. Obesity raises the risk of several malignancies, such as colon, esophageal, and kidney cancers. Consume a diversity of veggies, focusing on those that are dark green, red, and orange.

THE CANCER FIGHTING BREAKFAST

Natural folate is a crucial B vitamin that may help prevent malignancies of the breast, colon, and rectum. On the breakfast table, there is a ton of stuff. Good sources of folate include whole wheat products and breakfast cereals that have been fortified. Likewise, strawberries, melons, and orange juice.

MORE FOODS HIGH IN FOLATE

Asparagus and eggs are two additional excellent sources of folate. Additionally, it is present in legumes, sunflower seeds, and leafy greens like romaine lettuce and spinach. Not from a pill, but by eating enough fruits, vegetables, and items made with enriched grains, is the greatest method to obtain folate. In order to ensure that they obtain enough folic acid to help prevent some birth defects, women who are pregnant or may become pregnant should take a supplement.

TOMATOES THAT FIGHT CANCER

It's unclear whether the cause is lycopene, the ingredient that gives tomatoes their red color, or something else. However, some research suggests that consuming tomatoes may lessen your risk of developing certain cancers, including prostate cancer. Additionally, studies indicate that processed tomato products like juice, sauce, or paste have a higher capacity to fight cancer.

TEAS POTENTIAL TO FIGHT CANCER

Tea, especially green tea, may be a potent cancer fighter, albeit the evidence is currently fragmentary. Green tea has been shown to reduce or stop the growth of prostate, colon, liver, and breast cancer in laboratory experiments. Similar results were seen in skin and lung tissue as well. Additionally, in certain longer-term trials, tea consumption was linked to a reduced incidence of pancreatic, stomach, and bladder cancer. However, further human studies are required before tea can be suggested as a cancer preventative.

CANCER AND GRAPES

Resveratrol is found in grapes and grape juice, particularly in purple and red grapes. Strong anti-inflammatory and antioxidant effects are seen in resveratrol. In laboratory tests, it has stopped the type of cell damage that can start the cancerous process. The possibility that eating grapes, drinking grape juice or wine, or taking supplements can either prevent or treat cancer is not supported by sufficient data.

REDUCE ALCOHOL CONSUMPTION TO REDUCE THE RATE OF THE CANCER

Alcohol consumption has been associated with cancers of the mouth, throat, larynx, esophagus, liver, and breast. The risk of colon and rectum cancer may also increase with alcohol consumption. Although the American Cancer Society advises against drinking, if you do, try to keep your intake to no more than two drinks per day for males and one drink per day for women. According to their individual risk factors, women who are more likely to develop breast cancer may want to consult a doctor about how much alcohol, if any, is safe to consume.

PROTECTIVE EFFECTS OF WATER AND OTHER FLUIDS

In addition to quenching your thirst, water may also help prevent bladder cancer. Water dilutes the concentrations of probable cancer-causing chemicals in the bladder, lowering the risk. Additionally, you urinate more frequently when you drink more fluids. As a result, those substances come into contact with the bladder lining for a shorter period of time.

MIGHTY BEAN

Given how healthy beans are, it should come as no surprise that they may also aid in the fight against cancer. They include a number of powerful phytochemicals that might shield the body's cells from harm that could cause cancer. In the lab, these compounds inhibited tumor release of chemicals that harm neighboring cells and halted tumor growth.

CANCER AND THE CABBAGE FAMILY

Broccoli, cauliflower, cabbage, Brussels sprouts, bok choy, and kale are examples of cruciferous vegetables. These cabbage family members make fantastic stir-fries and can truly improve a salad. Most importantly, however, is that certain elements in these vegetables may support your body's defense mechanisms against malignancies like colon, breast, lung, and cervix. Although human trials have yielded mixed outcomes, laboratory research has proved promising.

LEAFY DARK GREEN VEGETABLES

Dark green leafy vegetables are rich in fiber, folate, and carotenoids. Examples include mustard greens, lettuce, kale, chicory, spinach, and chard. These vitamins and minerals may offer defense against stomach, skin, lung, larynx, mouth, and pancreatic cancer.

COOKING TECHNIQUES MATTER

The amount of cancer risk that meat carries can vary depending on how it is prepared. Meats that have been fried, grilled, or broiled at extremely high temperatures form compounds that may raise the risk of cancer. Stewing, braising, or steaming appear to produce less of those toxins than other cooking techniques. And when you simmer the meat, don't forget to include a lot of wholesome vegetables.

BLUEBERRIES FOR HEALTH

The strong antioxidants found in blueberries may be beneficial for many aspects of human health, beginning with cancer. By removing free radicals from the body before they can harm cells, antioxidants may help fight cancer. However, more study is required. To increase your intake of these beneficial berries, try adding blueberries to oatmeal, cold cereal, yogurt, or even salad.

AVOID THE SUGAR

Cancer may not be directly caused by sugar. However, it might replace other nutrient-rich foods that aid in cancer prevention. Additionally, it raises calorie intake, which plays a part in obesity and being overweight. Cancer risks can include being overweight. Fruit provides a healthy sweet alternative that is also vitamin-rich.

NEVER RELY SOLELY ON SUPPLEMENTS

Vitamins may aid in cancer prevention. However, that is when you naturally obtain them from meals. The American Cancer Society and the American Institute for Cancer Research both highlight that eating foods like nuts, fruits, and green leafy vegetables instead of taking supplements is by far the best way to obtain nutrients that prevent cancer. The best diet is one that is nutritious.

TOP 10 FOODS THAT FIGHT CANCER

1. Kale

It is scientifically proven that "Kale is one of my go-to options because it's rich in many phytonutrients like carotenoid-based antioxidants and other sulfur-based compounds, including indoles, which support natural liver detoxification processes, may help prevent DNA damage, or inhibit tumor blood vessel growth. Brussels sprouts, broccoli, cauliflower, arugula, and cabbage are other cruciferous vegetables. According to Kennedy, studies have shown that persons with diets high in certain veggies have decreased occurrences of specific diseases such stomach, prostate, and lung cancer.

2. Peaches (Apples)

According to studies, eating at least one apple every day may help lower the chance of developing malignancies of the breast, colon, lung, throat, and mouth. In addition to being delicious, apples also include quercetin, another antioxidant-based substance, fiber, and vitamin C. Kennedy advises choosing local and organic apples whenever feasible and eating them with the skin on because apples are on the EWG's Dirty Dozen Plus list. "Most of the nutrients are there," she said.

3.Tomatoes.

Tomatoes are an excellent food because they contain lycopene, a phytonutrient that has been linked to a lower risk of prostate cancer. When the tomato is cooked and has a healthy fat like olive oil or avocado, the lycopene is best absorbed, providing additional nutritional benefit.

4. Quinoa

A fantastic source of protein is quinoa (keen-wah). Because it has been grown for a very long time and is naturally gluten-free, it is frequently referred to as an ancient grain. Actually a seed, quinoa may be processed into flour. It is regarded as a complete protein, meaning that, like meat, it includes all nine essential amino acids. Quercitin, an antioxidant that we recently learned is also present in apple skin, as well as other phytonutrients like fiber and minerals like iron, magnesium, and calcium are all abundant in quinoa.

Quinoa is a tasty substitute for foods high in protein, such as meat and fish. Lentils, beans, nuts, seeds, and other whole grains are other substitutes.

5. Sweet potatoes

Other year-round foods include yams and sweet potatoes, despite the fact that they are not the same vegetable. They contain a lot of carotenoids, including beta- and alpha-carotenes, which are phytonutrients. According to scientific research, eating carotenoid-rich foods in even modest but regular doses may help lower the incidence of ovarian, lung, and breast cancer. Carrots, acorn or butternut squash, and pumpkin are additional foods high in carotenoids.

Research has it that supplements containing phytonutrients like carotenoids are available in it, but it cautions that these supplements lack the same preventive benefits as those found in whole foods and may even be harmful to certain people. Eating the meal rather than ingesting these supplements might not give you the healthiest boost.

6. Green tea can help prevent cancer.

Catechins, an antioxidant found in the leaves of the tea plant Camellia sinensis, may help prevent cancer in a number of ways, including preventing free radicals from harming cells. Tea catechins have been shown in laboratory experiments to shrink tumors and slow the proliferation of malignant cells. A few human studies, although not all, have connected drinking tea to a reduced risk of cancer. Both black and green teas include catechins, but green tea has a higher concentration of antioxidants, so you might want to include a cup or more of it daily in your anti-cancer diet.

7. **Turmeric May Lower Cancer Risk**

a dish of turmeric powder, which lowers the risk of cancer

This orange-colored spice, a mainstay in Indian curries, contains curcumin, a substance that is not the same as cumin and may be helpful in lowering the risk of cancer. The American Cancer Society claims that curcumin can prevent the growth of some cancer cells in lab experiments, halt the spread of cancer, or reduce tumor size in some animals. You may use this food, which fights cancer, in a variety of meals as part of your anti-cancer diet. It is simple to buy in grocery stores.

8.**Whole grain**.

Whole grains offer a variety of nutrients, such as fiber and antioxidants, that may reduce your chance of developing cancer, according to the American Institute for Cancer Research. More whole grains may reduce the incidence of colorectal cancer, according to a big study including close to 500,000 participants. As a result, whole grains are among the best diets to combat cancer. Whole grains include things like oatmeal, barley, brown rice, and whole-wheat bread and pasta.

9. **Red Grapes Can Help Prevent the Spread of Cancer Red grapes can help prevent the beginning or spread of cancer.**

Resveratrol, an antioxidant, is particularly abundant in the skin of red grapes. This antioxidant is also found in red wine and grape juice. The National Cancer Institute claims that resveratrol may help prevent the onset or development of cancer. According to laboratory tests, it prevents a variety of cancer cells from proliferating.

10. Beans That Fight Cancer Could Lower Your Cancer Risk
dried beans, which can lower the risk of cancer

Beans are frequently unfairly overlooked when discussing sources of antioxidants, although other fruits, vegetables, and other plant foods receive a lot of attention. You should include some beans in your anti-cancer diet since they are exceptional providers of antioxidants, especially pinto and red kidney beans. According to the American Cancer Society, beans also contain fiber, which may help lower your chance of developing cancer.

DEFUSING FEAR IN CANCER

It's normal to feel intimidated and frightened after receiving a cancer diagnosis because it can be an incredibly frightening experience. Here are some suggestions for easing cancer-related anxiety:

1. Learn more: Find out as much as you can about the diagnostic, available therapies, and prognosis of your cancer. You might experience less fear and more power as a result.

2. Consult your physician: Your doctor can inform you about your cancer, respond to your inquiries, and assist you in making choices about your course of treatment.

3. Join a support group or make connections with people who have gone through similar experiences to help you feel less alone and to give you a sense of community.

4. Self-care is important: Looking after your bodily, emotional, and mental needs can help you feel less anxious and afraid. Getting enough rest, maintaining a healthy diet, exercising, and practicing relaxation methods like deep breathing or meditation are some examples of how to do this.

5. Consider seeking professional assistance from a therapist or counselor if your fear and anxiety are affecting your everyday life.

6. Instead of worrying about the future, put your attention

on the here and now and accept each day as it comes. By doing this, anxiety and dread about the future may be lessened.

When receiving a cancer diagnosis, it's normal to feel scared and anxious, but there are things you can do to manage these emotions and feel more in charge. It's crucial to get the help you need from family members, medical experts, and mental health professionals.

LEARNING TO CHANGE IN CANCER

Learning to adjust while battling cancer can be difficult, but it can also be a great chance to reflect on your life and make progress. Here are some strategies for overcoming cancer:

1. Identify your priorities. Receiving a cancer prognosis can help you reevaluate your priorities and the things that matter most to you. Spend some time thinking about your priorities and any potential adjustments you want to make.

2. Accept self-care: During cancer treatment, it's critical to take good care of your bodily, emotional, and mental health. Getting enough rest, maintaining a healthy diet, exercising, and practicing relaxation methods like deep breathing or meditation are some examples of how to do this.

3. Seek support: Speaking with people who have gone through a comparable experience to yours can be a great way to get support and feel less alone. Think about signing up for a support group or making internet connections.

4. Learn new skills: If you're receiving therapy for cancer, you might need to pick up new abilities like how to handle side effects or deal with difficult emotions. Take advantage of these chances to improve and learn.

5. Make goals: Making realistic goals can give your cancer

therapy a sense of direction and purpose. This can involve both small objectives for self-care and bigger goals for your career or personal life.

6. Remain optimistic: Being upbeat can make it easier for you to handle the difficulties of cancer therapy. Try to discover happy moments throughout the day and concentrate on the things that make you happy.

7. Accept change: While receiving therapy for cancer may be a time of transition and uncertainty, it can also be a chance for personal development and transformation. Accept the changes brought on by cancer and use them as a chance for progress.

Keep in mind that learning to adjust while dealing with cancer is a process, so it's okay to move slowly. Be kind to yourself, get help when you need it, and concentrate on the life-improving adjustments you can make.

HOW TO PUT ON WEIGHT AFTER CANCER TREATMENT

One of the most crucial things you can do to lessen your risk of getting cancer and to increase cancer survivability is to maintain a healthy weight. But other people discover that their specific cancer or treatments cause them to lose weight, and they worry about how to gain it back following treatment.

Loss of appetite, taste alterations, and other symptoms that make eating challenging or unpleasant are frequent side effects of cancer treatment. Your metabolism may also be more "revved up" during this time, which could mean your body needs more calories than usual to maintain your weight. When you desire to eat less yet your body needs more food, it is simple to understand why you might be losing weight.

Nevertheless, there are measures you may take to stop excessive weight loss and encourage healthy weight gain throughout and after cancer treatment:

- Throughout the day, try to consume small, frequently spaced meals and snacks.
- To save your energy for eating, ask a friend or family member to assist you with food preparation and purchasing.
- Consider including calorie-dense, healthy foods like avocados and nut butters in your diet.
- Request that a relative or friend prepare a small cooler filled with easy-to-eat meals, healthy snacks, and liquids that you

can carry with you while you are sitting and resting or take with you when you are on the go.

- Your body need more calories, as well as more nutrients and protein. For the immune system, to combat fatigue, and to help maintain muscle growth, protein is crucial.
- Soups and smoothies are excellent providers of several nutrients and the essential water.
- Use smaller dishes and glasses because standard serving sizes can be intimidating.

THE WINNING MINDSET

A proactive and optimistic approach to cancer treatment and recovery is known as the "beat cancer mindset." The following are some crucial elements of the "beat cancer mindset":

1. Positivity: Keeping a positive outlook can help you get through the difficulties of cancer therapy and recovery. Try to discover happy moments throughout the day and concentrate on the things that make you happy.

2. Self-care: During cancer treatment, it's critical to take good care of your bodily, emotional, and mental health. Getting enough rest, maintaining a healthy diet, exercising, and practicing relaxation methods like deep breathing or meditation are some examples of how to do this.

3. Education and knowledge: Gaining knowledge about your cancer diagnosis, available treatments, and prognosis can make you feel more in charge and less afraid. This can involve consulting your physician, researching internet, and getting in touch with other cancer patients.

4. Social support: Talking to people who have gone through a comparable experience to you can give you much-needed encouragement and make you feel less alone. Think about signing up for a support group or making internet connections.

5. making goals: While receiving treatment for cancer and recovering from it, making realistic goals can give you a feeling of direction and purpose. This can involve both small objectives for self-care and bigger goals for your career or personal life.

6. Resilience and flexibility: While receiving treatment for cancer may be a time of change and uncertainty, it can also be a chance for personal development and transformation. Accept the changes brought on by cancer and use them as a chance for progress.

Keep in mind that the beat cancer mentality is about approaching the experience with a proactive and positive attitude rather than downplaying or denying the difficulties of cancer treatment and recovery. You can develop a mindset that aids in beating cancer and thriving in life by putting an emphasis on self-care, social support, information and education, goal setting, and resilience.

CONCLUSION

Uncontrolled growth and spread of abnormal cells define the complex and diverse group of diseases known as **CANCER**. It can affect any part of the body and is a major cause of death globally.

Despite the fact that the causes of cancer are complex and not fully understood, a number of risk factors have been identified, including environmental exposure to radiation and specific chemicals as well as lifestyle factors like alcohol and tobacco use, poor diet, and lack of physical activity.

Various treatment modalities, including surgery, radiation therapy, chemotherapy, targeted therapy, and immunotherapy, can be used to cure cancer. The sort, stage, and location of the cancer, as well as the patient's health and preferences, all influence the therapy option.

There are screening tests available for some kinds of cancer because early detection is essential to improving cancer outcomes.

It's essential to remember that there are no miracle treatments for cancer, and the success of a given course of treatment depends on a variety of variables, including the type and stage of the cancer, the patient's general health, and how well they respond to the treatment.

As a result, it's crucial to collaborate closely with a trained healthcare expert to create a thorough cancer treatment plan that is suited to your unique requirements and preferences. A healthy lifestyle, which includes not smoking, keeping a healthy weight, eating a balanced diet, exercising regularly, and getting regular checkups, can also lower the chance of getting cancer.

FURTHER READING

To learn more about cancer, check out these resources:

1. American Cancer Society: The American Cancer Society offers knowledge on preventing cancer and detecting it early, as well as information on therapy options and survivorship. Resources for caregivers, patients, and their relatives are also available on their website. (https://www.cancer.org/)

2. National Cancer Institute: The National Cancer Institute is a federal organization that disseminates knowledge about the causes, diagnosis, therapy, and prevention of cancer. In addition, they offer tools for doctors, nurses, and researchers. (https://www.cancer.gov/)

3. Mayo Clinic: The Mayo Clinic offers details on the signs, reasons, diagnosis, and treatments of cancer. Resources for cancer survivors and caretakers are also available on their website. (https://www.mayoclinic.org/diseases-conditions/cancer)

It's crucial to remember that these resources are only meant to provide knowledge and should not be used in place of seeking medical advice. Please seek the advice of an experienced healthcare provider if you have any concerns about cancer or any other medical problem.

AFTERWORD

Although battling cancer is never simple, it can also be a life-changing event that offers fresh perspectives on the human condition. The various facets of cancer have been covered in this work, from its causes and symptoms to its treatment and survival advice.

It's essential to keep in mind that there is hope despite the fact that receiving a cancer diagnosis can be terrifying and overwhelming. More and more people are surviving and thriving after receiving a cancer diagnosis thanks to novel therapies and treatments made possible by advancements in medical research.

Cancer patients and their families have access to a wide range of tools in addition to medical care. Throughout the cancer journey, support groups, counseling services, and other community-based initiatives can offer both emotional and practical support.

We must keep advancing our efforts to raise cancer awareness and prevent it, which is perhaps most essential. Cancer risk can be decreased by making healthy lifestyle decisions like consuming well, exercising frequently, and giving up tobacco. Regular cancer screenings can also aid in the early, most curable detection of the illness.

Please know that you are not fighting cancer alone if you are going through it right now. You have access to a sizable support network, and there is always optimism. And to those who have lost loved ones to cancer, we must keep paying tribute to their remembrance by striving for a time when receiving a diagnosis of cancer won't be as devastating.

I'd like to conclude by saying that I trust this book has given those who have been affected by cancer useful information and insights. Together, we can keep fighting this illness and strive to ensure that everyone has a healthier future.